FASTING, FEASTING, FREEDOM

A 33 Day Habit Creation Guide

WRITTEN BY KIM SMITH

An Unbelievable Freedom Book

Habit is a cable; we weave a thread of it each day, and at last, we cannot break it.

HORACE MANN

Table of Contents

Introduction

Greetings, Fellow Freedom Seeker. I'm Kim Smith, co-author of *Unbelievable Freedom,* a memoir named for the vibrant health and happiness experienced after adopting an intermittent fasting (IF) lifestyle in 2017. Ultimately, my husband Ryan and I have lost a combined 200 pounds in recent years. The IF process transformed us inside and out, and the memoir describes our entire journey with weight, food and diets. I went on to leave my job to promote the book and develop associated habit-creation products. I am a freedom enthusiast, and I have a strong desire to help others feel more freedom in their lives.

This brings me to the workbook you're holding (which I prefer to call a "Habit Creation Guide"): it originated as a 33-Day email mentoring series in late 2018. The Guide contains support and guidance to begin a journey of personal development based on a foundation of intermittent fasting.

Over the past few years, I've been transformed physically and mentally by making a series of significant behavioral changes, and daily fasting supports each one. I now live with radiant physical health and radical self-acceptance. The freedom I feel is so overwhelming that I feel compelled to teach others what I have learned.

Before we start, I am going to ask you to make one promise to yourself right now. I want you to put faith in yourself and your body. I want you to Believe in Unbelievable Freedom. Our beliefs are powerful, and our thoughts will make or break this process.

Your journey will be a personal one and its course depends on where you start from, but I believe committing to this 33-day program will launch you toward your goals.

The book was designed for readers to reflect on one daily message for 33 days, ideally in the morning as the day begins. The program is structured as follows:

Unit 1: Focus on Fasting (Day 1-11):

This unit covers topics related to the daily fast itself. My program is based on the concept of clean fasting as outlined in Gin Stephens' *Delay, Don't Deny: Living an Intermittent Fasting Lifestyle*. This was a life-changing book for me, and Gin has since become a mentor and friend. She reviewed and approved the content of the email series early on. These first 11 messages will support you in defining a fasting window and provide tips on dealing with hunger, coping with stress without food, etc

Unit 2: Focus on Feasting (Day 12-22):

This unit focuses on the daily eating window. There are no required or forbidden foods, but in this phase, you will identify the kinds and amounts of food that work the best for your body. We will unpack diet mentality thinking that may have been part of your old life. Optimal results will come from incorporating dense nutrition into your eating window, and your body's wisdom will lead the process.

Unit 3: Focus on Freedom (Day 23-33):

This unit focuses on the most important part, freedom. With "food noise" dialed down, you will create space in your life. I will provide guidance on how to turn the time and energy you've freed up into momentum for where you want to go next. I weave in information about practicing radical self-acceptance and gratitude, releasing limiting beliefs about your capability, and how to strategically pursue happiness as you define it.

Believe! See you in the morning!

DAY 1
Believe in Unbelievable Freedom

This Habit Creation Guide is a mix of directive information (do this, do that) and encouragement to trust yourself, your body and your intuition. You've probably been burned by diets that didn't work and tarnished your trust. We will be actively working to get in touch with your body's intuition and reject external diet rules.

I will refer throughout the program to this new "WOL", way of life, because IF, intermittent fasting, impacts far more than food. So, before we talk nuts and bolts, again, believe! Believe that you CAN implement these changes and they WILL make an incredible difference in your health and happiness.

Today, Day 1, we are going to do a 16-hour clean fast. What is a clean fast? It means abstaining from food for a prescribed time (sleeping time counts as fasting). Black coffee, black or green tea, or water (sparkling or still) are the approved beverages. More later about why clean fasting is so important to keep insulin levels low and create the "appetite correction" you need to become a successful intermittent faster. If you're like me, the clean fast will make all the difference in your success. It sounds impossible, but it isn't - it is challenging but do-able, and each clean fast builds your fasting skill set.

Don't worry about when you last ate yesterday; just focus on today. After your fast, the eating window will be 8 hours long. I'm going to use example times since you all have different lifestyles and obligations to meet. For example purposes, this will be an eating window of 10:00 AM - 6:00 PM. If your life requires it, flex this time earlier or later, but stick to 8 hours. 9:00A-5:00P is fine. So is 12:00P-8:00P. Some use an app like Window or Vora to track their fasts; many just keep an eye on the clock (that's what I do).

Inside your eating window, eat what you want. You'll be hungry when your window opens, but listen to your body and eat what it asks for. For most people, this will mean two meals and possibly, a snack in between. Don't restrict anything based on your old diet unless it's something you don't tolerate. Once your eating window "closes", you are back into the next day's fast.

The first few days are the hardest. Remember that fasting is a skill for life and one that takes practice. Be flexible as feelings and sensations arise. Be patient with yourself and the process. And most importantly.....

Believe in unbelievable freedom....

Kim

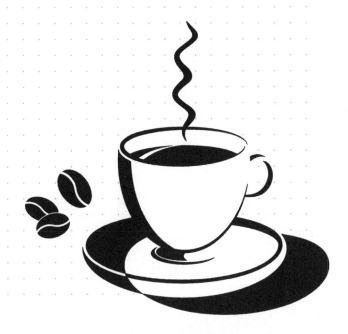

DAY 2
The Transformation has Begun

Good morning! You're reading this with your first clean fast under your belt. Congratulations. Take a minute and pat yourself on the back. It's good practice for the radical self-love and acceptance attitude that will fortify your fasting lifestyle as you proceed. If things didn't go as planned, leave it in the past. Every day is sparkly, shiny new fast.

Depending on your history with eating and dieting, you may have found the fast difficult or you may have breezed through. In either case, today may be different. Some struggle Day 1-2 and then sail smoothly, others find it easy for the first few and then hit a wall where the fast feels tough. That's why this is a 33-day program. The support and encouragement will continue as you experience the first critical weeks of your journey.

We are still on an 8-hour eating window, so your timeline should be much like yesterday. You will clean fast outside the window, then eat as you wish within it. Reflect on yesterday - do you feel you ate enough, or not? Some people who've dieted long term have a hard time giving themselves permission not to count calories, so be patient with yourself if you're among them. You don't need to count calories because the clean fast itself is healing your metabolism. The further you go in this process, the easier it will be to know just what your body wants and how much. So eat to satiety, and enjoy! It's not just fasting, it's about feasting.

Tomorrow, we will talk specifically about black coffee. If you already take it that way, it may not be an issue for you. For many, it's the one sticking point that keeps their fast from being clean. I can tell you as a long-term creamy coffee drinker, now that I clean fast consistently, I keenly feel how a sip of coffee with cream breaks my fasted state like a snapping twig. It's why I believe in and promote the clean fast so strongly...more on that in the morning!

Believe in unbelievable freedom....

Kim

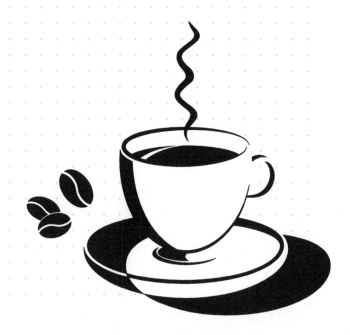

The Blacker The Coffee

Good morning!

Here you are on Day 3. Some of you found yesterday harder than Day One. Others of you may have found it easier. Each day is a new fast and there is a lot of dynamic stuff happening "behind the scenes." Your body is now adapting to a period of digestive rest daily, a time during which its resources are not focused on a big influx of food, but instead are devoted to healing. Increasing evidence is showing that a clean fast helps speed up a process of "autophagy", which is how cells break down their unused parts and regenerate themselves. This is why IF has anti-aging effects - it helps the metabolism, the immune system, the health of the gut, and so much more!

How do we keep our fast clean? Gin Stephens' book *Delay, Don't Deny: Living an Intermittent Fasting Lifestyle* gets into this in detail, but in short, it's by having NOTHING during the fasting window except plain coffee, tea, and water. No broth, no juice, no mints or gum, nothing. This prevents the body from secreting insulin, healing underlying insulin resistance and correcting the appetite by balancing hunger hormones.

In our coffee-obsessed culture, the biggest sticking point is usually folks and their love of creamy, sweetened coffee. If you enjoy morning coffee, the transition to black coffee will make a huge difference in your progress. You have two options: taper down on the sweetener, then creamer OR rip off the band-aid. I recommend option 2. It seems scary (there's a section in our book *Unbelievable Freedom* devoted to my fear) but as with so many things in life, it's never as bad as it seems. Pour that black coffee and take a sip. Shudder if you have to. Each day it will get easier, and most people come to find they love black coffee after the initial adjustment.

Adapting to black coffee will give you a beverage to count on and even look forward to during fasting. If you don't like coffee at all, it's not necessary. Stick with black or green tea, or just water. The clean fast is supposed to be boring! There will be plenty of excitement when that fasting window opens!

Believe in unbelievable freedom.....

Kim

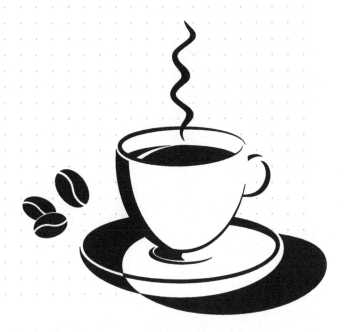

Tweaking the Tastebuds

Hey! It is Day 4! That means you're over halfway through the first week of your fasting journey. I hope you've had some moments of feeling pretty proud of this change. I say fasting makes me feel "rugged" and nearly three years in, I have those moments of rugged pride.

If you consumed your first cup of black coffee, extra kudos for that. Even though millions around the world do it daily, it's a big step and a big change for us who live in the land of a million sweet, flavored creamers. Drinking black coffee is a huge step for your palate. Some find that drinking a light roast helps. Some find that using cold brew iced coffee, which is less acidic, helps ease the transition. Whatever it takes to get you into a black coffee routine, the benefits make it worthwhile. I believe that adjusting to black coffee creates a big impact with helping your taste buds stop seeking sweet.

Yes, eating sweets within your eating window is absolutely allowed. BUT, trending away from sweet will create more space to eat nutrient-dense food, which supports your journey toward better health. My deep cravings for sugar and starch quieted from fasting itself, but black coffee also helped my tastebuds. Bathing the palate in something bitter offsets the baseline preference for sweet. Despite numerous advantages to a black coffee routine, IF is about enjoying your life, so give it a few weeks and if it's not getting better, let it go.

When you break your fast, whether it's a meal or a snack, pay attention to the kinds of foods your body is really asking for. This will gradually shift as your palate does. You will find foods you used to love don't taste the same anymore, and that is a normal part of the process.

For today: keep your 16-hour clean fast (with or without black coffee) and eat what you want in your 8-hour eating window! You're doing it!

Believe in unbelievable freedom…..

Kim

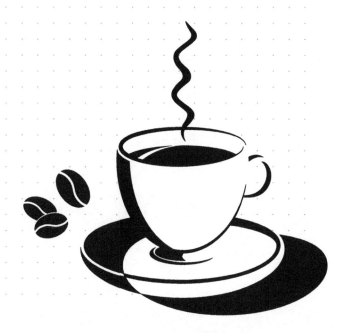

Hunger is Not an Emergency

Hello! Day 5 is here and today we are going to talk about HUNGER. I know, you've experienced a lot of it over the past few days, but I still think this may come as a newsflash: Hunger is NOT an emergency! Many diet mentality mantras in the past have been about eating frequently to keep the metabolism from "shutting down" and as such, the first wave of hunger sets us out to find some sort of healthy snack to tamp down that hunger pang. That may be an actual sensation in your stomach getting your attention, and eating will (briefly) quell it. You know what else will quell it? Just waiting a little bit. I get sensations of stomach hunger for a few minutes here and there during the morning/early afternoon, and I ignore them entirely. I don't tune into them, they don't cause me stress, and they go away.

Another thing that happens is that sad/stressful moments trigger a desire to eat for the soothing effect food has. Makes perfect sense, and it's how I spent decades of my life coping with emotions. One big lesson of my intermittent fasting journey is that hunger will come and go just like ocean tides - so will waves of emotion.

When you don't numb an emotional reaction with a sudden influx of food, you have to FEEL it, and you'll be amazed at how emotions move through without becoming a big deal. Take a breath, take a walk, cope with the emotions without food, and feel empowered! You have absolutely got this.

Are there times when hunger becomes intense and you need to eat no matter what the clock says? Yes, absolutely. In every step of this journey, you have to listen to your body, and there are times it will tell you it needs food. You and your body are on the same team. So, eat, have your eating window even if it's a longer one, and start again the next day. This is a flexible lifestyle without a need for any sense of failure.

Believe in unbelievable freedom.....

Kim

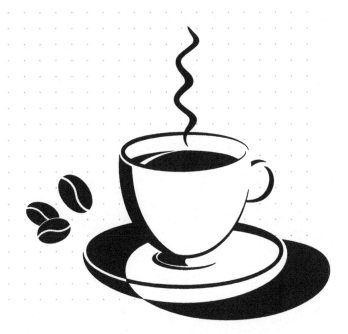

Let's Talk About the Scale

I haven't mentioned it yet, but I am not a scale fan. For the bulk of my IF journey, I weighed myself just once a month. That's right, 30 days, no scale. It took off so much pressure and helped me really judge my progress based on how I felt, how I looked in the mirror, and how my clothes felt. However, I realize I am an exception to the rule and that most of you have probably gotten on the scale once or twice (if not daily).

Here is why the scale is especially tricky when you are embarking on an IF journey: IF, unlike other diets, creates dramatic body recomposition. There are people who do IF and drop an entire dress size without the scale budging an ounce. Fasting increases human growth hormone, which can build muscle mass and may even slightly increase bone mass. Therefore, you can be having dramatic results behind the scenes of your body's inner workings and the scale won't give you one iota of validation.

So, it's a personal decision. The thing to remember is what I said at the outset: this journey will be a success if you believe, have faith, have patience and persistence. You are almost a week in and I've heard over and over, "I got on the scale, it hasn't budged. I fasted all week and nothing happened! I'm done!" This short-sighted attitude makes me so sad. If I had quit after a week, I would have missed out on so many life-changing health benefits that IF has brought to my life.

Gin's advice is that if you must weigh daily, keep track and compute a weekly average. Over time, you will see a downward trend even if it is not readily apparent day to day. Some apps will do this for you automatically.

It's a marathon, not a sprint, so focus on your long-term transformation. Remember, you do this process one fast at a time, and the weight will eventually come off, one pound at a time.

Believe in unbelievable freedom.....

Kim

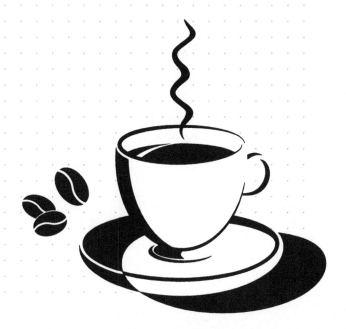

DAY 7
Breaking Fast (Early)

And here it is, the day that marks the end of your first week of fasting. This is a milestone to be celebrated...with a cup of black coffee or another clean-fast-approved beverage! I hope you're feeling the first hints that this lifestyle is going to work for you. Sometimes it takes as little as a week for people to note a decrease in inflammation, bloating, and other subtle symptoms that show the body is healing through their daily fasts.

I want to talk some more about the decision to open the eating window earlier than planned. This is a decision that can trip people up. I've already advised that hunger is not an emergency and thus you should distract, stay busy, push through, tough it out, several variations on that theme. But what about the times when your body gives off a stronger signal?

You're only a few days into this process, but you will learn to know the difference between the annoying and distracting stomach grumbles that come and go, and the body truly sending a distress signal that it needs food. I can't explain why, but even with abundant fat available for burning, there are still days when the body needs food. It doesn't happen often, but there are still days it happens to me, and I've been strictly clean fasting going on three years.

My strategy for dealing with this is simple: I drink some water, give it 10-15 minutes and if the hunger is not abating, I eat. Yes, you've broken your fast, but every day is a new day and a new fast. It's nothing to beat yourself up about or to feel significantly disappointed over. If it works for your life, close the window early since you've opened it early. If you have a special dinner planned later on, just have a window that's longer than 8 hours today. It is not a big deal. I promise!

Flexibility and patience are key traits necessary to succeed. It's why I encourage people to stay off the scale. The healing is gradual and body recomposition cannot show in frank numbers. Your clothes and the mirror will tell you more. There's nothing I hate more than someone who tells me "I did IF for two weeks then quit because the scale said I didn't lose anything." IF is a marathon, not a sprint, and you stand to gain way more than a medal at the end.

Believe in unbelievable freedom......

Kim

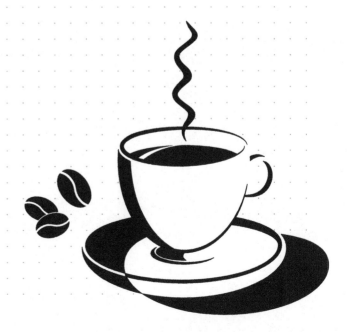

DAY 8
Coping Without Food

Here we are in Week 2, so let's talk about coping without food. I am guessing that many people who have chosen to undertake an IF lifestyle have some history of struggles around food, and that is often linked to using food as a stress reliever or source of emotional comfort. SO, what do you do if you are fasting with several hours to go and those emotions flare up? Stress, anger, sadness...how do you cope if you cannot reach in a desk drawer for chocolate or run for some starchy carbs?

I've written on my blog about emotional numbing with food. As per the disclaimer at the outset, this course is not focused on the clinical treatment of disordered eating, but even those of us without a diagnosis have fallen prey to the temptation to eat until we have "numbed out" of the emotional state we sought to avoid. The problem with eating to avoid feelings is that you don't face them. You prolong the inevitable.

The number one most empowering part of my IF journey is the way that I've learned that I am capable. Capable of not eating, yes, but also capable of facing those tough feelings head-on with nothing but myself. To breathe, to move, to let the feelings come and go like waves washing up on a beach. Every single time you do it, you get stronger. In my online communities, I've heard it again and again. Sit with the feeling (or walk, run, dance with the feeling) but cope without food and it's amazing. Like hunger waves, the stress/sad/disappointed/frustrated waves will also pass. You have the power.

Keep this in mind as we prepare to increase the fast and decrease the eating window in a couple of days. You've got this!

Believe in unbelievable freedom....

Kim

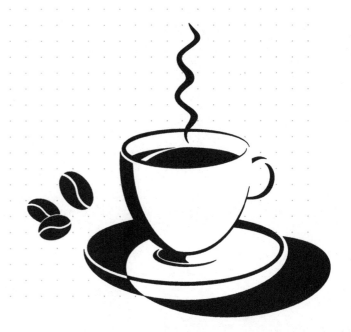

DAY 9
Oops, I Botched My Fast

Good morning, it's Day 9 of the first 11 days focused on fasting. I hope that most of your fasts have gone smoothly. Progress, not perfection. Sometimes a clean fast is less than squeaky clean. Sometimes you set out for a 16-hour fast and it ends up being not quite that long. But what about when you botch it completely? Wake up, decide to eat breakfast, intend to close early, but the next thing you know, you ate from sun up until sundown?

It's OK. Days like this happen. I hope for your sake that one hasn't occurred yet, but even if it hasn't, it may. This is where the mindset piece comes in: you need to develop a fasting mindset, one that says, I'm already into my next fast. Leave what is in the past behind and focus on getting right back into that fasted state.

Your body is very forgiving. How many diets have you been on? I'm asking rhetorically, but I suspect your answer is a high number, maybe even an honest "I don't remember, but too many to count." I'm asking you to view this new way of life as distinctly different from any of those diets in the past. This is not a diet that you can mess up or fail. This is not a start-over-again Monday. In a fasting mindset, fasting is something we do every day for the sake of our health. We do it to give our body space to rest from digestion and focus on other important tasks like regeneration, rejuvenation, and breaking down inflammation and toxins.

Try to take the negative words out of your vocabulary. Yes, I said "BOTCH" in the title, but fasting isn't something you can botch, fail or flub. It's just a new part of your life that you do without self-judgment. You don't botch your sleep, you don't botch your breathing, so let fasting be as natural to you as those activities are.

And speaking of negativity, tomorrow we'll talk about what to do when it's directed at you from others.

Believe in unbelievable freedom......

Kim

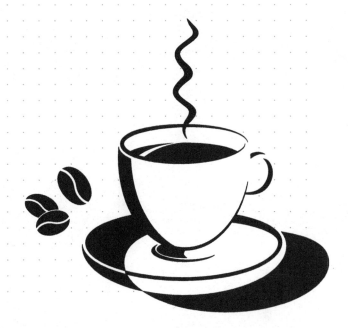

Dealing with Negative Nellies

Let's be real - there is pushback when you majorly change your way of life, especially if your new way doesn't jive with other people's old ways. Here we are on Day 10 and you've likely encountered someone who is skeptical or even sabotaging.

From my blog in the early months of my journey, with regard to the steely resolve I felt (and feel) around IF as a personal conviction for my life:

Everyone else's opinions don't matter.

If you are a woman. A mom who has not put herself first in many years. Or if you are wired to be a people pleaser, an approval seeker. Supremely conflict avoidant. If you are naturally neurotic or overthinking. If you have a tendency to be easily swayed by others or, as Charlie Brown was called, you are (or have acted) just plain "wishy washy."

Or if you are me and just checked All of the Above. THIS is the transformational, revolutionary part. Everyone else's opinions don't matter. I have found this thing, it works beautifully for me and I don't need your approval. I don't need to know if you think it is weird. Doesn't matter what information you have to the contrary. I'll still be polite, that's still who I am....but I DON'T CARE about your opinion.

And then it starts to spill over into so much more than food & eating

Do I think you should necessarily be there already? No, but hear what I am saying: you are doing this for yourself, to create transformation and find freedom. You can be gentle and patient with the naysayers, but do not let them knock you off your course. You chose this path for a reason, and you are doing this for your health, because you deserve it!

Believe in unbelievable freedom....

Kim

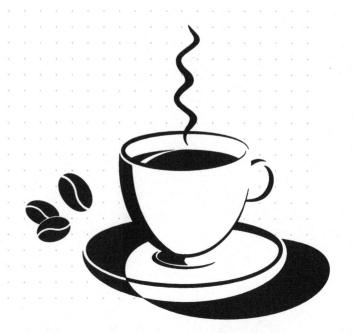

Day 11
Unit 1 is Complete!

And just like that, here we are on Day 11, and you are completing Unit 1 of my program. Today is the day when make the first increase of the fasting window (or decrease of the eating window; they offset each other). I suggest that you accomplish this by shaving a half hour off either end. If you have been doing a 10:00-6:00 eating window, make it 10:30-5:30. If it's not practical to get your eating window closed by 5:30 due to work schedules or other reasons, make it 11:00-6:00. In terms of the way you talk about your IF regimen, you will now be doing what is known as a "17:7", 17 hours of fasting and 7 hours of eating.

It is possible that some of you have had this happen organically. Perhaps you just haven't felt hungry at the time you're scheduled to open, so you've been pushing it a bit further. For the purpose of guiding the process, I've chosen Day 11 as the time to shave off an hour. If you've been doing this a bit more gradually, that's fine too.

This is the chance to practice all the skills you've been building over 11 days: remembering that hunger isn't an emergency, using a little extra black coffee, green tea or additional water. Stay busy, another fasted hour will pass, and you'll become even more adapted to burning fat for fuel instead of food. In time, instead of distracting, you'll embrace the hunger pangs as signs of your body's digestive rest and clean up. Congratulations on reaching the end of the first Unit. Tomorrow, we begin our Focus on Feasting.

Believe in unbelievable freedom.....

Kim

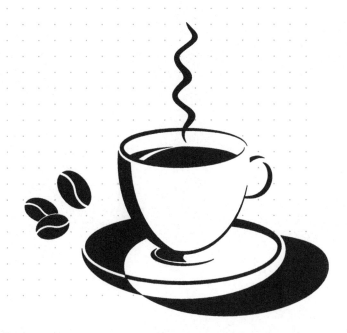

Day 12
Break the Fast Right

Welcome to Unit 2, Focus on Feasting! Of course, you've been feasting daily all along, but now we spend the next 11 days focusing in on the eating part of the fasting/feasting contrast. Today I want to talk about how you break your fast, what you've been choosing to "open your window."

It's been a learning process, but I have found the right balance of fat and protein to open my window. In the beginning, I opened with sweets, but over time, my body no longer asked for that. I tend to open with nuts (cashews, almonds, pistachios) or with Perfect Bar, which is a refrigerated nut butter based protein bar, or with cheese or avocado. I sometimes eat high protein oatmeal with chia and quinoa. What works for each person is based on their individual physiology, but I want to stress that making the right choice for your body is important.

You want to get your digestive system up and running in a way that's gentle and comfortable. You don't want to cause gastric distress right after a nice period of digestive calm and quiet.

You want to choose foods with a lot of nutrient value. The body has been in a nutrition deprived state (focused on its own internal workings) and it's primed to uptake nutrition readily. There is even a theory that the brain starts to associate the taste of the foods you use to "open" with the rapid uptake of nutrients, thus creating an affinity for those particular foods. So if you have a food you know is good for your body and you want to love/crave it even more, using it as a "window opener" can help cement that process.

Tomorrow we'll talk about OMAD vs. TMAD and some of the philosophical parts of planning your feasting window. Some of it is semantics, but I'll give guidance on how to think about your feast and talk about it when you (inevitably) are asked by others about this new thing you're doing!

Believe in unbelievable freedom....

Kim

*****

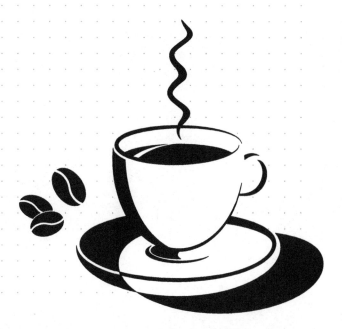

OMAD VS TMAD

A huge buzzword or term in the IF community is "OMAD", which stands for one meal a day. That's where agreement on the subject stops. Some people who say they follow an OMAD lifestyle mean they eat one plate of food a day, whether lunch or dinner, one meal they sit down to, and then they are back to fasting. This often equates to a 23:1 fasting regimen. The contrast to that would be TMAD, or two meals a day, for people who eat what they call lunch, wait a few hours, then eat dinner. With or without snacks involved, eating two distinct meals is called TMAD.

For the bulk of my fasting journey, I've eaten what I call OMAD. As with so many things, I take my cues from Gin Stephens and her *Delay, Don't Deny* lifestyle. Gin eats one meal that sometimes starts with a small appetizer or snack while cooking, progresses to a leisurely meal, then may extend to dessert or after-dinner cocktail. She consumes all of this within 4-ish hours. This is exactly how I eat, and I often say my regimen is 19:5 or 20:4. The numbers get confusing, but the philosophy is the same: eating the equivalent of one large, multi-course meal extended over enough time to enjoy it, but also enough time to get 20 hours of fasting in daily.

For this 33-day program, you are still on a 17:7 regimen and likely eating two meals (TMAD), which is great. Your body may lead you to condense that considerably as time goes on (and a few days from now, this program will direct you to condense it down a bit, as the goal at the end of our 33 days is to have you at an 18:6).

Happy feasting!

Believe in unbelievable freedom....

Kim

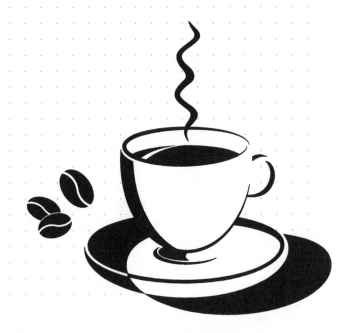

Day 14
Do You Really Like Your "Favorite" Foods?

Let me be clear: Fasting has completely changed my tastes, and I believe the strong cues I receive about what my body wants and needs have helped to optimize my nutrition. This optimal nutrition, along with fasting, has created the radical transformation in my body that inspired this entire program.

Vegetables: the range of vegetables I find tasty has widened, and even more so, the fact that I crave vegetables daily and don't feel satisfied if I haven't had them, that is new.

My consumption of organic, grass-fed dairy has increased, while my overall intake of meat has decreased to nearly none. I went from being a daily meat eater, to 1-2 servings per week, and I suspect I'm headed for vegetarianism.

There is a theory that listening to the specific nutrition your body is asking for will create deeper satisfaction overall, which makes fasting easier and more effective, so get invested in figuring out what you REALLY like, not what you think you like. This means starting to filter out old triggers (too many M&M cookies because they remind me of Gram) and external messages like other people's food desires, advertising and societal messaging, etc.

It turns out that most everything I thought I liked, mostly inexpensive processed food like Kraft Mac & cheese and Pop-tarts....I don't like at all. And I like greens, beans and grains, all previous 'yuck' foods, more than I ever knew. Will your experiences or changes mirror these? Only time will tell.

Believe in unbelievable freedom....

Kim

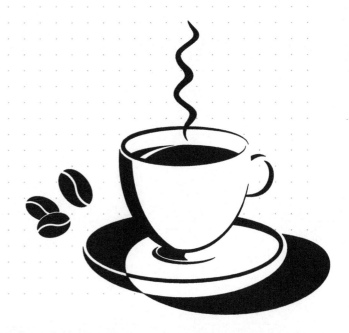

Day 15
Have a Plan-Structured Yet Flexible

Good morning! It is Day 15, do you know what that means? You just finished Week 2 and are heading into Week 3. You aren't quite halfway through my 33-day program, but today you will be halfway through the magic 30 day number that is often discussed when talking about habit creation.

So let's talk about what it means to design your feasting window. Those who have read *Delay, Don't Deny*, sometimes use the phrase, "I can eat anything I want." This is a reference to the fact that indeed, the program has no forbidden foods. In theory, you may eat a large pizza and a half gallon of ice cream in your window every single day. Are those optimal choices for weight loss or even for overall health? Probably not.

As your appetite corrects, your body only has room to accept so much total food each day, so it's best to find a way to fit in mostly nutrient-dense food with good fat, protein, vitamins and minerals AND a bit of those things that are really enjoyable and keep you from feeling deprived. I accomplish this by having a plan that I call "structured yet flexible." I eat one snack and one meal each day. Sometimes the snack is small (a protein bar like Perfect Bar, a packet of nuts). Sometimes the snack is large, like a plate with salami, cheese, olives, pita chips, nuts,etc. Many would call that a light meal, but if it's what I feel that I want, I have it.

When I eat dinner, my actual MEAL, I have a plan, too. We eat from the meal kit services or buy/plan meals that involve one large portion per person. There aren't seconds to deal with. Almost all of the time, this plate of food is plenty, but if it doesn't seem like enough, I add an avocado, an extra serving of dairy, or I may eat a bigger dessert.

Thus, my eating window is not chiseled in stone, nor is it a 4-hour food free-for-all. I encourage you to consider the same. Have a general plan with some boundaries, and let your body drive a bit of flexibility about your portions, etc.

Believe in unbelievable freedom....

Kim

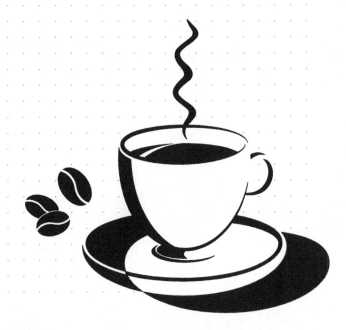

Day 16
What Happens When You Eat Too Little?

Good morning! Today, I want to talk about a subject that creates a lot of confusion for people in their initial weeks of an IF journey. What happens when you eat too little? Especially when people have a lot of weight to lose, it's natural to wonder how there can be such a thing as eating too little. After all, aren't we teaching our bodies to burn fat for fuel? Isn't there plenty of excess fat available for use? There is even a famous story in the literature of an obese person who fasted for an entire year (under medical supervision) while consuming no food whatsoever!

Yet, I believe for each of us, there is such a thing as eating too little. It's hard to give you specifics, which makes it uncomfortable for those who have been on rigid diets with rules. Many people who've been on a restrictive diet such as low carb, low fat or calorie counting, may inadvertently take those habits into their IF life. If you let those limits carry over, you are giving your body a double whammy: you are putting it through fasting (a good stress on the body) AND also putting it through the restriction of not much fat, very few carbs, or very little food overall.

I can't specifically say for any given person whether this down-shifts the metabolism, but I look at the IF lifestyle holistically. You're trying to work with your body so that it trusts that lots of wholesome food is coming in following each fast, and so you feel emotionally and psychologically satisfied. I'm careful to eat foods that make me most satisfied - starchy vegetables like sweet potatoes, beans and lentils, and moderate fat in the form of olive oil, butter, avocado, nuts, and full-fat dairy. This has kept me satisfied through my daily fasts.

It may feel scary to eat lots of food, especially ones you've restricted, but you can do so and still lose weight. This is what clean fasting accomplishes for the metabolism. So when you are fasting, fast....and when you are feasting, FEAST. Eat plenty of fat, protein and a reasonable portion of carbs, preferably unrefined ones, plus little treats here and there. Your body will let you know what it needs as you get better and better at listening to its cues.

Believe in unbelievable freedom.....

Kim

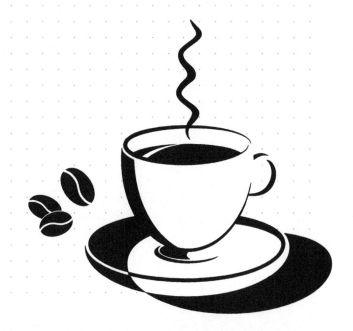

Day 17
What happens when you eat too much?

Yesterday we talked about what happens when you eat too little: the impact this can have on you psychologically in terms of feeling deprived, as well as the risk of the metabolism getting a double whammy from fasting plus limited food. So today, we'll flip the coin and talk about eating too much.

What is too much? I wish I could give you some kind of concrete amount. If you have read Gin Stephens' *Delay, Don't Deny* (and I hope you have), you know that you're allowed "whatever you want" in your eating window. Gin has clarified this to mean foods that agree with your particular body, but you still have a responsibility to figure out what those are. This topic still creates turmoil and controversy ....you mean, WHATEVER I want? Double cheeseburgers? Candy? Half a lasagna? A whole bottle of wine? Technically, as long as you delay until your eating window opens, you may have these things and be following the plan.

However, we are trying to create something called Appetite Correction or "AC." I'm no authority on AC, but there are many resources out there, including a book by Dr. Bert Herring that is exclusively written on the topic. The idea, in a nutshell, is that the combination of daily fasting and eating to your actual hunger/satiety cues work in harmony so that the appetite is driven by what the body needs on a given day. You'll likely have very hungry days, and barely hungry days.

If you are constantly eating based on what your eyes want, what your emotions want, or what the people around you want, it will be harder to achieve AC. It will still happen gradually if you are fasting daily, but you can streamline the process by listening to your body and eating enough, but not too much. You CAN do it! It's a trial-and-error process that evolves each day.

If you want pizza, have a slice or two, not six. If you want ice cream, have a scoop, but not an entire pint. You may have already noticed how much more quickly you feel full. If you have not noted a dramatic change, that effect may still be on its way, but it is coming soon. Don't push against it. Notice it and let it guide you to eat the amount that's perfect for the lifestyle you're designing.

Believe in unbelievable freedom....

Kim

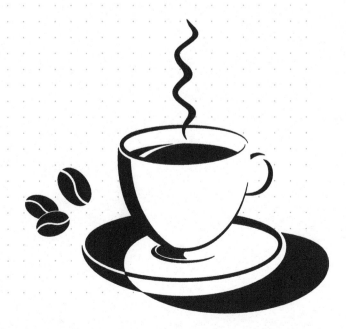

Day 18
The Joy of Cooking

The past week has been spent focusing on the feasting window portion of the day. For those following this program exactly, that's the 7-hour window in which you eat vs. the 17 hours during which you fast. We've looked at our changing tastes and a bit about being intentional not to eat "too little" or "too much", which varies for each of us.

Now I want to talk about food preparation. Depending on individual/family situations, you may or may not have had a dramatic change in your food-related responsibilities since beginning an IF journey. Because our children are grown, Ryan and I are down to just planning/prepping 7 meals a week. This has transformed meal preparation from a major chore to (mostly) a pleasure. Even if you've got loved ones to cook for 21 times a week, I hope the space created by fasting is helping you see the work of handling food with a new attitude.

We do use meal kits like Plated and Home Chef a few nights a week, which simplifies and streamlines things, but we also make meals from scratch. We love to make soups, stews, and casseroles. The real joy comes from anticipating each meal as an event, as something that only happens once a day (we eat one snack/one meal).

We are more intentional about our food choices, and we enjoy being in the kitchen getting the food ready for the meal we are going to sit down and mindfully enjoy. Some of the food we eat is simple, but it's all prepared for maximum nutrition and enjoyment. We like to say, we've come a long way from Shake & Bake and Rice-A-Roni every night.

Have you been enjoying food prep or cooking in a different way? I hope so. If not, try to shift your mindset around it. Look at it as less of a chore and more of a joy. It's all done in the service of your ongoing health transformation.

Believe in unbelievable freedom.....

Kim

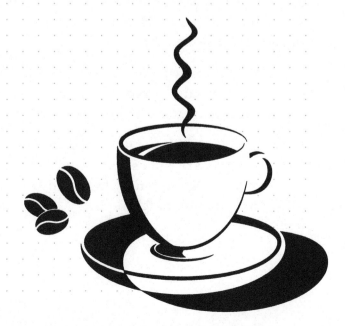

Day 19
What Does Kim Eat?

We're moving toward the end of the third week of this process. Amazing! 19 days ago, you might have questioned whether you could do 19 clean fasts in a row.

Soon, we shall once again extend the fast by collapsing the eating window. In the meantime, you are keeping a 17:7 for now. That's a longer eating window than I personally keep at this advanced stage in my journey (I eat for 3-5 hours daily, week in and week out). But once my window opens, what DO I eat?

A frequently asked question I get asked is "What does a day's food look like for you?" Because that question came up over and over, I began a ritual of posting photographs of my food several times a week. It's a tradition I continue to this day. So, here's what a typical day looks like for me.

3:00 PM - A latte or creamy coffee with a Perfect Bar or rough-cut oatmeal with chia seeds, nuts and dried fruit (that's the sweet 'opener' variation). Perfect Bars are organic nut-butter based bars found in the refrigerated section in many grocery stores. They are uniquely satisfying for me, and a great item to open my window because they're substantial enough to tide me over 2-3 hours until dinner. This is how I open my window at least 4-5 times a week.

If I'm home with Ryan, especially in the summer, I might have a plate of olives, cheese, hummus and chips, and a few pistachios or cashews (the savory 'opener' variation). A lot of times I drink kombucha with this snack. It works the same way; it's substantial enough and gets my system up and running to be ready for the big evening meal to come.

5:30-6:00 PM: My dinner. This is often something from a meal kit OR our own version of the same....occasionally chicken or salmon, more often beans and roasted vegetables, sometimes potato or rice, and occasionally bread. We add a salad a couple times a week. If it is from a meal kit service, it's one big plate of food. If we make it at home, seconds are an option, but I rarely feel like I want them. Full appetite correction means that I am very satisfied with the plate I make and sit down with.

6:30 PM: We close with a hot beverage (decaf coffee and cream, hot chai latte, golden milk made from turmeric, cardamom, and honey) and some squares of dark chocolate. Sometimes full-fat yogurt with honey, and sometimes, especially if I didn't open with one: a Perfect Bar.

I'm Kim and this is how I eat. These are just examples of the way one person eats for IF success. The variations are endless, and what matters most is what will make your body feel great, will fuel you through your next fast, and what makes your psyche feel you're eating abundantly and deprived of nothing!

Believe in unbelievable freedom....

Kim

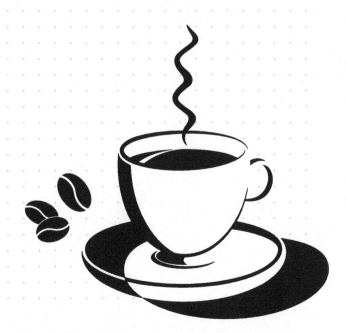

Day 20
Intuitive Eating Demystified

I'm not sure if any of you had curiosity about the Intuitive Eating movement over the years, but I sure did. I read many books on the subject and everything about it resonated with me - working with your body, listening to its cues, eating when you are truly hungry and stopping when you are full. I wanted to learn to be an intuitive eater. The fact that it sounded so simple and remained so difficult felt like a huge failure, one I beat myself up over.

You know what turned me into an intuitive eater? Intermittent fasting. I am convinced that for some of us, we reach a point where physiological barriers disrupt our ability to be intuitive with our bodies. This is likely tied to insulin resistance and the role it plays in our appetites, though I can't explain the science precisely. I only know that a big I.E. question was, "What is your body asking for?" and my body always asked me for chocolate chip cookies and donuts. Always.

In your new life as an intermittent faster, your clean fasts are healing your metabolism, your insulin regulation and your hunger hormones. This dials down the volume of food noise, and in that calm and quiet, you will be able to hear what your body actually wants. It's amazing and wonderful. Sometimes mine wants an avocado and sometimes it wants salmon and sometimes it wants pistachios. It usually wants a serving of full-fat dairy in the form of grass fed milk or high quality cheese or yogurt. It almost always wants Perfect Bars.

Some ask, isn't it "counterintuitive" to say that you get hungry during your fast and don't eat? Strict I.E. teaches eating when hungry as a way of working with your body. I understand my hunger cues and the ones I ignore are not truly my body needing to eat. It's my stomach doing its fasted thing - when it's really time to eat - I eat and enjoy, and I stop when I am full. Just like I.E. always taught that I could.

Believe in unbelievable freedom...

Kim

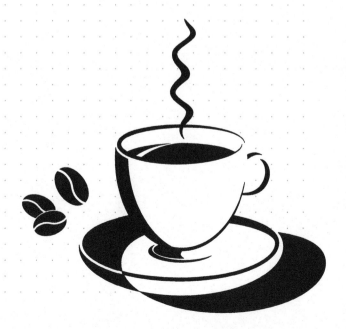

Day 21
Fearless Feasting

You all know that I am a big fan of the work of Gin Stephens, and I've referenced *Delay, Don't Deny: Living an Intermittent Fasting Lifestyle* multiple times. Its the book that "started it all" and I feel like it is the how-to book for how I live. But, it has a companion, and that title is *Feast Without Fear*, also by Gin Stephens. FWF was published in October 2017 when I was a little over four months into my IF journey. I was already having success, and felt clean fasting was clicking for me, but the book was well-timed in terms of its message: find the foods that work for YOU, eat the way YOUR body wants to eat. It highlights how we are all different in terms of our ancestry, so there is no reason to expect that the exact same foods are right for or will agree with all of our bodies.

The thing I love about the book, aside from Gin's accessible presentation of information about food and cultures around the world, is how it reinforces the message of what IF is about for me: individuality and empowerment. Eating meat may be wrong for one and right for another. Have you heard about "lectins"? These are certain plant proteins that don't agree with certain people, but I eat lots of lectin-heavy foods, which tend to be rich in many other nutrients as well. The same applies to dairy. The same applies to gluten. The same applies to incorporating or eliminating sweets, processed foods, etc.

The central message of the book is that food is shift your thinking from food being bad or good, to food being right or wrong FOR YOU. This will allow you to enjoy food without guilt and without falling into traps created by outside authorities dictating what you should eat. Certainly we should listen to the latest scientific findings, but those also change rapidly like shifting sands, so listen to your body. It knows what it needs and it wants to be radiantly healthy.

Believe in unbelievable freedom....

Kim

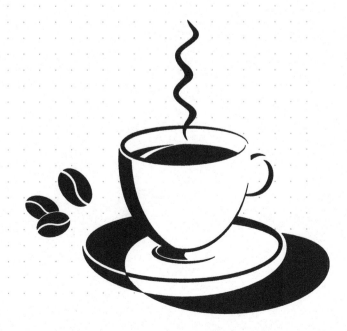

Day 22
Unit 2 is Complete!

Here we are Day 22, at the end of Unit 2: Focus on Feasting! Now, part of your focus will remain on your daily feasts forevermore, but tomorrow, we are going to shift the focus to Unit 3: Focus on Freedom. I'm so excited to start guiding you through some of my thoughts on how Intermittent Fasting can change your life beyond your relationship with food and eating. I have experienced truly Unbelievable Freedom through this way of living, and though I can't convey it all in 11 days, I look forward to sharing some of the highlights.

This is also the second time in our time together that we are going to increase the fasting window/decrease the feasting window. Today is the day we go to 18:6, or 18 hours of fasting with 6 hours of eating. Some of you may have done this already, others may have been waiting for the cue but welcome it, and others may read these words with dread. I genuinely believe the health benefits mean everyone should try to do their eating within 6 hours, and it is especially important if you have goals around weight loss.

If you have been doing the 11:00-6:00, today is the day to go to 12:00-6:00. Like last time, you could shave a half hour of either end, and go to 11:30-5:30. Again, the evenings are the trickiest time because folks who work need time to get home from work and get the meal prepared, eaten, etc. Even a 12:30-6:30 could be a decent window. Don't be rigid about getting it timed down to the minute, but make it your goal to start eating within an approximately six-hour window daily.

Congratulations on coming this far. It has only been 22 days, but I hope your life is already changing in tangible ways.

Believe in unbelievable freedom....

Kim

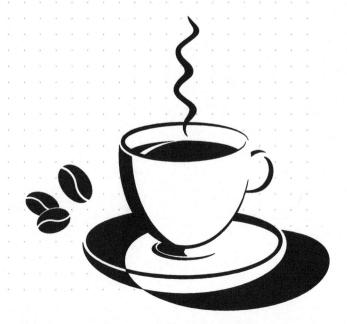

Day 23
The Freedom Formula

Now we reach the part of the program that is closest to my heart, Focus on Freedom. For the final 11 days of the program, we will be talking about what I consider to be my Freedom Formula of sorts, the ingredients in the recipe that have combined to give me success far beyond the improvements in my physical health.

The formula is a combination of mindset work (positive thinking, letting go of old limiting beliefs, taking action instead of staying stuck), what I consider broadly to be spirituality (gratitude, self-acceptance, recognizing your own gifts and uniqueness) and movement (walking, dancing, being in nature, finding things that bring you joy).

Each day of the 11 will have a theme with my thoughts and suggestions on what worked for me and what might work for you as you expand from freedom with food to more freedom in your life broadly. There are several days when I will make a suggestion of a book I've read that helped me or informed my thinking, but there is no required reading list. I will give you enough info that you can benefit without investing time or money in books (unless you want to do so).

I've been saying it from Day One, but over this next stretch, it really is time to get excited. Yes, Intermittent Fasting is a regimen for timing your eating, but it's so much more. It will change your life if you let it. Center your thinking around this, how do I want my life to feel when I've reached my IF goals?

Believe in unbelievable freedom....

Kim

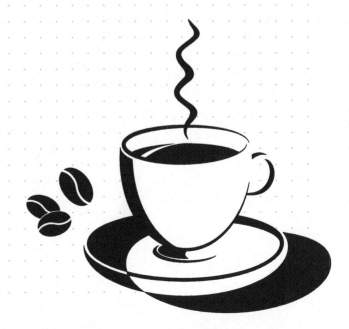

Day 24
Radical Autonomy

Today I'm going to talk about what I call Radical Autonomy. I ask myself if it's "too soon" to go there with all the personal empowerment stuff, but you've been reading my messages for 24 days now. You get my vibe, and you continue to follow the path with me. So let's talk about what it really means to PUT YOURSELF FIRST, to trust yourself, to in essence be your own best friend. It is a shift in mindset that will help frame the rest of our time together.

Even in our culture (I'm talking American culture, though there may be a few reading who aren't Americans), which is one of supposed rugged individualism, it's still a radical act to non-conform. As I talked about in Unit 1, "Dealing with Negative Nellies", there are going to be times when you decide that you are going to fast through an event, even if other people don't like it. You are going to adhere to this new way of living even when criticism is lobbed at you or worse, people deliberately try to sabotage you.

Each time this happens, it moves you into a place of Radical Autonomy. You are truly putting yourself first in terms of your body and how you take care of it. It moves you into that mythical place where you and your body are "on the same team", so to speak, and it lays the groundwork for you and your mind to get on the same team. Quiet the self-criticism, turn down the negative self-talk, and start being your own best advocate and friend in all areas of life.

It's a MAJOR mindset shift for most of us, so I'm not pretending you read one message and undo years of mental habits, but keep this in the front of your mind as we proceed: You're the one who is in charge of your body and your life. When you start living from that mindset, you start to feel really empowered to make other kinds of decisions in your own best interests. Even better, others around you begin to respect and even emulate your new attitude in time. Self-care isn't selfish, and being radically self-focused is part of what frees you.

Believe in unbelievable freedom....

Kim

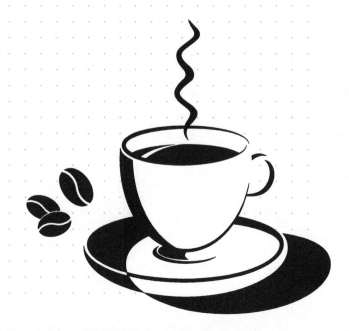

Day 25
Investing Your Savings

Hard to believe, but here we are on Day 25 - cruising toward the end of the first month of your intermittent fasting journey. Hopefully, you are doing well with your new 18:6 regimen. The extra hour of fasting is undoubtedly increasing the benefits your body is getting from extra autophagy, and likely fat burning with associated body recomposition is happening, too. But what else are these longer fasts creating?

There are two tangible categories of savings compared to your pre-fasting life: you are saving TIME and you are saving MONEY. Fewer meals each week means less time thinking about food, buying food, preparing food, and even eating food. We don't think of the time it takes to eat as significant (many of eating way too quickly or on the run), but it still adds up in the course of a week. This saves you mental energy along the way, too.

The financial savings will depend greatly on how you eat, but it's hard for there not to be some kind of savings of money when you go from 21 meals to 14 or 7 (7 plus snacks = how I eat). We do buy higher quality produce, dairy, coffee than we used to, and this offsets some of the cost savings, but we do save overall. If you've read our book, you know we've always lived on a budget, so this has been a huge benefit to our lives.

What will you do with the saved time and saved money? If you tune and focus on it, you will see how it creates a sense of increased freedom. My real passion for IF is the way it creates SPACE. There is a place in your life where all the food struggle used to be, and within that space is huge potential to do, feel and be what you've always wanted to be. We will talk more about this in the days ahead.

Believe in unbelievable freedom...

Kim

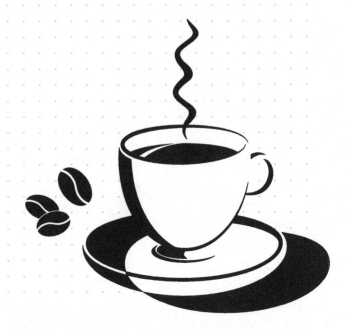

Day 26
Embracing new routines

We talked a bit already about "investing" the savings of your new-found time. For many people, the change to an IF lifestyle from their old way of living has created very specific pockets of time. You may have 15 minutes where you used to prepare/eat breakfast (or sit in a drive-thru line!). Depending on how you are structuring our current 17:7 regimen, for example, if you are doing a mid-afternoon snack/mini meal plus a later dinner (2PM-9PM, say), you might have found yourself with 30 minutes around noontime where you previously ate a more traditional lunch.

Time is a precious commodity, so when you find yourself with a little pocket of it, it's a gift and one that can directly contribute to the growing sense of freedom. But what do you DO with it?

For me, one example of a new routine is the walking regimen I embraced with my 30 minutes of "non-lunch" lunch break. Because I knew I did not want to eat, I needed something else to do. Even though I can be around people who are eating during my fast and it doesn't bother me in a temptation sense, I chose to embrace a new routine. Walking during my workday. It was simple

I made the walk something lovely to look forward to - walking in the fasted state, feeling centered but energetic, really noticing the scenery. I started walking in a historic neighborhood near the hospital where I work. So much landscaping! So many cool architectural details! I often say, IF has turned my life into a bit of a moving meditation. Everything is in sharper focus.

This is what worked for me. What new routine might you embrace? It depends on what you did in your old life and what you might want to build into the new. The options are endless, but aim for something you look forward to more than the eating you used to do in that space.

Believe in unbelievable freedom....

Kim

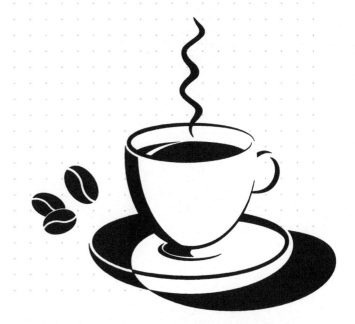

Day 27
Practicing Intentional Gratitude

Was anyone an Oprah fan back in the day? Of course, many of us were! In addition to being famous for her talk show and her weight fluctuations, Oprah's the first person I remember discussing gratitude as a practice. She is the first one who talked about gratitude as something you DO, and since then, an industry has sprung up around gratitude journals, gratitude calendars, gratitude jars, etc.

At the time, I remember finding the whole concept a little out there, but it's now how I live. Gratitude as an intentional practice has changed my life as a specific part of releasing my old narratives. I used to tell myself I was a person meant to struggle. Over the past few years, as I've become more intentional about gratitude in all situations, I've become exquisitely attuned to my blessings.

This is not specific to my weight loss. This part of my journey came before IF, and I think it helped me get into a mindset where I saw how much good I already had and how much more I deserved. The more blessed I feel, the more blessings I see, and the cycle repeats. I have a wall hanging above my bed that says #blessed, because it's truly how I feel.

A specific example is my morning shower. Each day when I step under the stream of hot water, I think about all the people who do not get a hot shower every day. I reflect on people who are homeless and don't have access to a shower. I even think about the millions of people who lived and died before technology made hot baths an accessible luxury. And because of this reflection, I start my day deeply grateful. Not everyone looks at the world the way I do, but everyone can start to tune in to the abundance of goodness around them.

I feel blessed by my family, my friends, my health, the beauty of other people and the natural world. Most of all, I feel grateful for the Unbelievable Freedom that I enjoy through my intermittent fasting lifestyle. I hope you are feeling it, too.

Believe in unbelievable freedom...

Kim

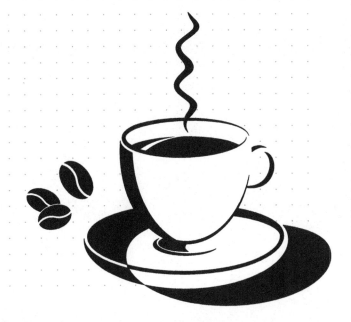

Day 28
Staying Action-Oriented

One of the keys to success in an Intermittent Fasting lifestyle is being action-oriented. Fasting itself is an active process. Some may view it as the absence of action - not eating - but fasting is a state of being where you are actively choosing not to eat to support a process inside your body. This is not a passive thing, but an hour-to-hour decision to move away from food and toward other activities so your body can rejuvenate and regenerate.

If you have read our memoir *Unbelievable Freedom*, you know that there was a moment where I poured my black coffee and started to drink it, like ripping off a band-aid. This was truly an active decision, one that is the same as standing at the end of a diving board and deciding to jump. I often wonder how my life would be different now if I had made a different decision, if I had poured the black coffee down the sink or scooted over to the fridge to slosh a ton of cream into the cup. If I hadn't actively embraced clean fasting, where would I be now?

In my travels on social media, I am a Top Fan of Mel Robbins on Facebook and I'm often found recommending her book *The 5-Second Rule*. If you are fasting and you are near food that's tempting you to eat....5-4-3-2-1 walk away from it. If you are sitting on the couch and you planned to exercise, you can't wait for inspiration to strike, you just 5-4-3-2-1 get up and grab your shoes. This sounds overly simplistic, but it's so empowering when you realize that you can outsmart your brain and its ability to get overemotional/overthinking and just MOVE. It is a game-changer if you've often found yourself stuck.

The most direct application of the 5-Second rule in my own life is 5-4-3-2-1 getting out of bed when my alarm goes off. No snooze button. After years of hitting snooze multiple times, the rule has helped me break that habit and I now get up earlier and feel more rested. This allows me to ease into my day more mindfully and intentionally. Freedom from the snooze button is part of the freedom.

Believe in unbelievable freedom....

Kim

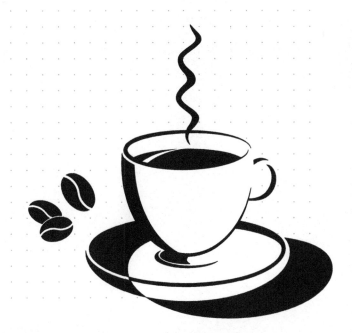

Immunity Against Perfectionism

Hard to believe but tomorrow will mark a month that you've been at this. I'm so proud of you and happy for you. You've made the commitment that will make it much more difficult to turn back to your old ways of frequent eating.

But let's talk about today's topic, perfection/imperfection. Are you a perfectionist? It took me a long time to come to terms with it, but I was. I talk about this in my sections of our book Unbelievable Freedom, especially when discussing my childhood. There was a feeling of shame that came over me when I felt someone would look directly at me and see me as less strong, graceful, smart or capable than someone else. This caused me to freeze up and to avoid certain activities, especially athletic ones. It drove me to focus on the things I felt I could do well, and mostly those were my academic studies.

This same type of perfectionism, ironically, let me to eventually tip that scales at more than 100 lbs over my ideal weight. The feeling of failing at diet after diet, the torture of never seeming to "get it right", it all caused me to shut down and give up. I could have avoided a lot of mistery if I'd figured out a way to recognize my perfectionism and how the pressure I put on myself was toxic, not motivating or productive.

Radical self-acceptance has given me a layer of immunity against perfectionism. We've talked a little bit about this earlier in the Freedom unit. I see myself as a kind, thoughtful person who works hard to encourage others, and I don't need to get my eating (or anything else) "perfect." Good enough is good enough, and I strive to simply take care of my body and enjoy my life. It's a far more peaceful way to live.

For more on this very important topic, I recommend *The Gifts of Imperfection* by Brene Brown. It contains tons of powerful insights about shame, vulnerability, and the freedom that comes from self-acceptance and self-worth.

Believe in unbelievable freedom...

Kim

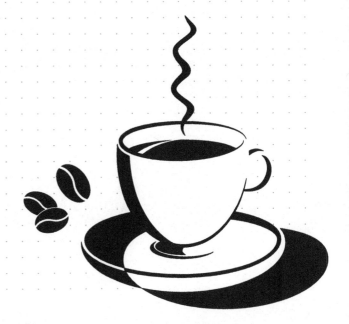

Day 30
ULP!

Good morning! Today I want to talk to you about The Upper Limit Problem, or ULP. If you've seen my recommended reading list, you might recognize that this comes from a book called *The Big Leap* by Dr. Gay Hendricks. It's an interesting little book that talks about how we all have an internal thermostat for just how happy we think we should be or deserve to be. This has been hardwired into us going all the way back to our childhoods. We don't think about it consciously, but it comes into play when things in our lives start going really well.

Because feeling really happy might not match what we think we deserve, we can subconsciously engage in behaviors that trip us up and bring the "temperature" back to where we feel it belongs. This is sometimes called self-sabotage, and all can fall prey to it. This is especially relevant when we are making health-related lifestyle changes like transitioning to an intermittent fasting lifestyle. We start to feel really good, maybe our weight starts to move downward, and it's all so unfamiliar and in a way, uncomfortable.

It's an important thing to be mindful of because we can absolutely self-sabotage. You might find you are pushing your eating window longer than planned many days in a row. You may find yourself moving backward into eating kinds or amounts of foods that remind you of the old days. Every slip-up or less-than-stellar moment with food doesn't have to be classified as an ULP, but be mindful and intentional. ULPing has happened to me, and it could happen to you, too.

As with everything, the freedom comes from being flexible, enjoying the process, and looking at this new skill of fasting as one that takes practice, yet will serve you forever. That thermostat Dr. Hendricks references can be permanently reset, and you can invite in all the health and happiness in the world.

Believe in unbelievable freedom...

Kim

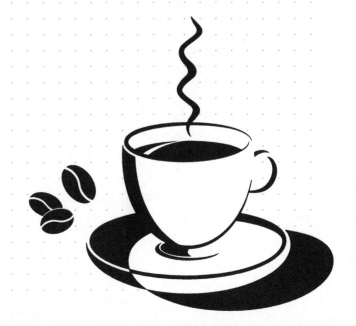

Day 31
Release Old Narratives

Here you are, into your second month of your IF life and just a couple of days from finishing my program. You may have previously told yourself a story about how you are not somebody who can go 18 hours a day without eating, but now, with perhaps an occasional exception, you are doing it! Negating or letting go of an old story can be a systematic process of proving yourself wrong in something you have long said as self-talk. Intermittent fasting is a great way to prove to yourself that you are capable.

Many people who've had long histories of struggling on a diets carry a story about themselves that they are weak-willed or undisciplined around food. A major breakthrough that happens when clean fasting heals the metabolism and balances out insulin & hunger hormones is the realization that it wasn't about willpower. There was actually something about your old lifestyle and old way of eating that fueled that constant drive to eat. Letting go of a story about yourself as weak-willed will empower you to make other positive changes in your life.

A few months ago, I dabbled with running. It was mostly taking my pace up for short sprints while out on walks, but I was running. I started to proudly proclaim, "I'm a runner! I run, so I'm a runner." As a person who had never been athletic or graceful, this was a powerful thing to claim. One day I was running along the river near our house and I thought of myself as a scared, small child who never felt capable or strong. It's hard to describe, but in a moment, I felt "her" leave my body. That old narrative about myself was actually released in a moment, like a weight lifting off me. It was something I'd carried and no longer needed to haul. And since then, I've chosen to do that more intentionally with other things.

What old stories do you tell yourself about your worth, your abilities, your values? It is worth examining in a systematic way. The language matters, too. It's why I reject anyone saying they can't drink black coffee. They may choose not to, but we all CAN do that and most anything we set our minds to doing.

Believe in unbelievable freedom...

Kim

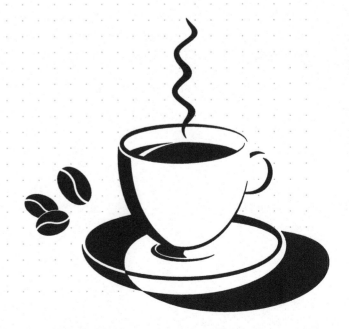

Day 32
My Ideal Day in the Future

At this time tomorrow, you will have completed my entire 33-day program. I'm so happy for you and the freedom you are already feeling, and all the good that is to come. You are continuing to do your 18:6 with an 18-hour clean fast and a 6-hour window feasting on foods that allow you to take care of your body and enjoy your life.

So now I want to ask you, what is your long-buried dream? As the months ahead unfold, some of the things you once wanted will begin to resurface. You dreamed your dreams for a reason, and even though life often gets us super sidetracked, they are right there waiting when we are ready to tune back in. We've talked a lot about saving time and money with IF, and now, we shift our attention to something deeper.

Years ago, when I was in graduate school studying to be a career counselor, we used a guided imagery exercise called, "My Ideal Day In The Future." In the exercise, clients were guided through an imaginary day in their future from start to finish. What time do you want to wake up? What do you wear? Where do you head first? What kind of work do you do? What type of people are you surrounded by?

I always loved the idea that you could design your life to feel exactly like you want it to feel. One person wants to wake up early and head outdoors, spend the day in solitude doing physical work. Another wants to sleep in, then head to a crowded space to work guiding tours in a busy museum. Every single one of us has strong preferences for how we spend our time, who we spend it with, and what kind of physical environment we spend it in. Sometimes we need only make tiny tweaks to our current reality. Sometimes we need an entire life overhaul. Either one gets achieved a single step at a time.

So today, on the eve of completion of this 33 day Habit Creation program, I invite you to think about your long-buried dream. Think about the day you have ahead of you today, and what would need to change for it to look like your "ideal day" from the exercise. Transformation isn't all physical, but it's all possible.

Believe in unbelievable freedom...

Kim

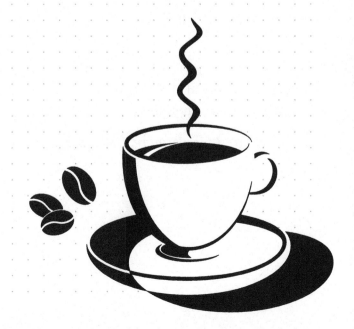

The Freedom Habit is Created!

Congratulations! You have completed the program. Surely there have been moments over the past 33 days that have not gone exactly as planned, but that's OK. Flexible and forgiving are themes you will carry forward. You have to be patient with yourself, and adaptable in terms of how you make IF fit your life, both in the way it looks now and the way it will look in the future. These 33 days were just the beginning of what I hope is a whole new practice that you'll use to improve the rest of your life.

I want to close today talking about ALL THE FEELS. Whether or not you've been getting on and off the scale, whether or not the fit of your clothes has changed dramatically, you know how you felt 33 days ago, you know how you feel right now, and most of all, you know how you want to feel in the future. If you're feeling like your mind is clearer, your energy level is higher, you've reduced your inflammation or bloating, the quality of your sleep is better.....these are all wonderful, expected responses. The way to continue to feel that way is to continue living your IF lifestyle.

Everything I do in my life now is driven by THE FEELS. When I extend my fast an extra hour, it's because it makes me feel good. When I break my fast early to drink a beautiful espresso latte, it's because it makes me feel good. When I accept or politely reject food that's being offered, it's because of how it makes me feel. When I decide whether or not to eat seconds or go for dessert, I use the same barometer. The same for spending time with, the same for distancing myself from negative people. The same for taking a walk, going out dancing, singing karaoke, sitting by the river.....whatever I do is because it makes me feel good.

As for your fasting/feasting regimen, I encourage you to treat it as an ongoing experiment. Some will stick at 18:6 long term. Others will quickly condense to 19:5 or 20:4 (maybe even have already). For some, the answer may be going back to 16:8, temporarily or permanently. We all have such different physical realities and need to continue to craft an IF regimen to fit ourselves.

You only have one body and one life, so figure out exactly how you want to feel and build everything else around that. If you feel like you want to continue this conversation with me, check out my newest guide, Poster Girl Habits: Guided Contentment Practice, coming late 2019.

And now and forevermore, believe in unbelievable freedom!

Kim

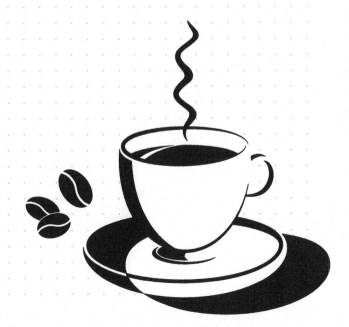

Made in the USA
Coppell, TX
03 November 2022